Simplified Solution Approach
To BELL'S PALSY

Unlocking Facial Resilience: A Comprehensive Guide to Restoring Vibrant Health and Reclaiming Your Radiant Smile

Dr QUENTIN GLYN

Table Of Contents

CHAPTER ONE
Bell's Palsy

Bell's palsy is a neurological condition that affects the facial nerves, causing one side of the face to suddenly become paralyzed or weak. Bell's palsy is named after the Scottish physician Sir Charles Bell, who first reported it in the 1800s.

Bell's palsy may strike anybody at any age and is often a transient ailment. It is essential to comprehend this illness in order to have a prompt diagnosis and suitable therapy. The goal of this book is to close the information gap and provide those who are dealing with Bell's palsy with a more approachable approach to managing this difficult disease.

An Outline Of Bell's Palsy

Definition: When the facial nerve (cranial nerve VII) malfunctions, it may cause a transient kind of facial paralysis known as Bell's Palsy. Although the precise etiology is often unclear, viral infections—specifically, the herpes simplex virus—are thought to be a contributing factor. This condition impairs taste, tear production, and facial emotions by causing abrupt weakening or drooping on one side of the face.

The prevalence and incidence of Bell's palsy are comparable, with 20 out of every

100,000 individuals affected by the condition each year. Although it may happen at any age, the most typical age range for it is 15 to 60. Although the precise etiology is yet unknown, it may occur as a result of viral infections, diabetes, respiratory infections, and familial history.

Early Diagnosis And Treatment Are Critical

Early identification and therapy are critical for Bell's Palsy sufferers. Early intervention may help control related symptoms and greatly increase the likelihood of a complete recovery. It is essential to get medical assistance as soon as possible in order to rule out other possible reasons for facial paralysis, such as stroke, and to start the proper therapy, which may include corticosteroids.

Prompt diagnosis also helps avoid consequences, such as problems with the eyes. Bell's palsy sufferers may find it difficult to close their afflicted eye, which may cause dryness and possible injury due to facial muscular weakness. These issues may be avoided with appropriate care, which may include using an eye patch or artificial tears.

The Objective Of The Book

1. Closing the Knowledge Gap: By offering concise and understandable information, this book seeks to close the knowledge gap about Bell's Palsy. Many people may

experience feelings of being overwhelmed and confused over the disease and its consequences after obtaining a diagnosis. The goal of this book is to provide patients and their families with the knowledge necessary to deal with the difficulties related to Bell's palsy by providing the material in an understandable way.

2. Empowering People with Bell's Palsy: Knowledge is simply one aspect of empowerment; another is receiving helpful advice. The book will include information on coping strategies, lifestyle modifications, and recovery-promoting activities. Along with offering support and encouragement to people who are dealing with facial paralysis, it will also address the psychological and emotional components of the illness.

To sum up, this book is a thorough resource for anybody coping with Bell's palsy and presents a solution-focused approach that highlights the significance of prompt diagnosis, suitable treatment, and the empowerment of those impacted. The book aims to enhance the general well-being and quality of life for those coping with Bell's palsy by demystifying the illness and offering helpful suggestions.

CHAPTER TWO
Knowledge Of Bell's Palsy

A neurological disorder called Bell's Palsy is characterized by the abrupt development of facial muscular weakness or paralysis, usually affecting one side of the face. It bears Sir Charles Bell's name, a Scottish physician who first reported the ailment in the 1800s. Although the precise origin of Bell's palsy is unknown, viral infections—specifically, the herpes simplex virus—are thought to have a role.

The Facial Nerve's Anatomy:
The seventh cranial nerve (CN VII), sometimes referred to as the face nerve, is

an essential part of the peripheral nervous system. It starts in the brainstem and spreads to the different facial muscles. The facial nerve transmits taste sensations from the anterior two-thirds of the tongue and regulates the muscles involved in making facial emotions.

The Functions Of The Facial Nerve:

The face nerve serves both sensory and motor purposes. Controlling the muscles that produce facial emotions like smiling, blinking, and eyebrow lifting is referred to as motor function. The sensation of taste for the front two-thirds of the tongue is one of the senses. The facial nerve also contributes to the production of tears and saliva.

The Pathogenesis Of Bell's Palsy:

Although the precise origin of Bell's palsy is still unknown, viral infections—specifically, the herpes simplex virus—are often linked to the condition. Bell's palsy is thought to be caused by viral inflammation, compression, and swelling of the facial nerve inside the fallopian canal, a tiny bone tube through which it flows. The inflammatory reaction impairs the nerve's functionality, which results in the recognizable paralysis or weakening of the face.

Symptoms And Indications:

Paralysis or Weakness of the Face:

The abrupt development of weakness or paralysis on one side of the face is the primary sign of Bell's palsy. The afflicted person may find it difficult to grin or shut their eye on that side as a result.

Taste Loss:

The anterior two-thirds of the tongue provides taste signals via the facial nerve as well. As a result, Bell's Palsy may cause the afflicted side to lose or change their flavor.

Additional Correlated Symptoms:

Eye issues: Bell's palsy may cause excessive tearing, ptosis, or drooping of the eyelid, as well as light sensitivity in the afflicted eye.

Greater Tear Production: Some people with Bell's Palsy may notice greater tearing on the afflicted side since the facial nerve is involved in tear production.

Drooling: Some people may find it difficult to regulate their saliva and may drool as a result of impairments to the muscles that govern saliva.

Hypersensitivity to Sound in One Ear: Bell's Palsy is seldom linked to an elevated level of sound sensitivity in one ear.

Early Diagnosis:

Early intervention depends on the symptoms being identified as soon as possible. When facial weakness or paralysis is seen, it is imperative to seek medical assistance.

Medical Assessment

A medical expert will do a comprehensive examination, evaluating facial expressions, taste perception, and other relevant processes.

Using Corticosteroids:

Prednisone is one of the corticosteroids that are often administered to treat inflammation and aid in healing. Early initiation of therapy is linked to greater results.

Eye Health:

It is essential to protect the injured eye in order to avoid complications such as corneal abrasions. This may include using lubricating eye drops and sleeping with an eye patch on.

Physical Medicine:

During the healing process, physical therapy may help to preserve muscle tone and strengthen the muscles in the face.

Continuation Care:

It is crucial to follow up with medical professionals on a regular basis to assess any residual symptoms and track development.

To sum up, Bell's Palsy is a disorder that affects the facial nerve and may cause abrupt paralysis or weakening in the face. Comprehending the structure, operations, and pathophysiology of the facial nerve is crucial for streamlining the diagnostic and treatment process. For those with Bell's palsy, early medical intervention—including corticosteroid medication and supportive care—can greatly improve prognosis.

CHAPTER THREE

How To Diagnose Bell's Palsy

Clinical Assessment:

1. Evaluation of Face Weaknesses:

• Sudden onset facial weakness, generally on one side of the face, is the defining feature of Bell's palsy. Doctors assess the extent and pattern of weakness in the muscles of the lips, eyes, and forehead.

2. Eye Exam

• It's important to evaluate the patient's ability to shut their afflicted eye completely since some Bell's palsy patients may have trouble doing so, which may cause dryness and irritation in the eyes.

3. Taste Perception:

• Taste alterations are possible for some people, especially in the front two-thirds of the tongue. This may be evaluated throughout the course of the test.

4. Tear Formation:

Bell's palsy may impair tear gland function, thus screening for dry eyes and excessive tear production is crucial.

Diagnostic Differentiation:

A comprehensive differential diagnosis is necessary since a number of illnesses may produce facial weakness. Other possible reasons for facial paralysis include of:

• A stroke

• Lyme illness

• Hunt syndrome by Ramsey

• Compression of the facial nerve due to tumor

Diagnostic Examinations:

Imaging Research:

1. Magnetic Resonance Imaging, or MRI:

• To rule out other possible reasons for facial paralysis, such as tumors or strokes, a head MRI may be conducted.

2. Computerized Tomography (CT) scan:

• To rule out other potential reasons and get comprehensive pictures of the structures within the skull, a CT scan may be advised in certain circumstances.

EMG, Or Electromyography:

1. Studies on Nerve Conduction and EMG:

Electromyography is a technique used to assess muscle electrical activity. Studies on nerve conduction evaluate the face nerve's capacity to carry electrical signals. The location and degree of nerve injury may be ascertained with the use of these tests.

Blood Examinations:

1. Studies on viruses and Lyme disease:

• Since viral diseases like the herpes simplex virus and Lyme disease may sometimes result in facial paralysis, blood tests may be performed to screen for these conditions.

Puncture Of The Lumbar Region:

1. Analysis of Cerebrospinal Fluid:

• To check for indications of inflammation or infection in the cerebrospinal fluid, a lumbar puncture, often known as a spinal tap, may be advised in some situations.

In summary:

A mix of clinical assessment and diagnostic testing is used in a complete approach to Bell's palsy diagnosis. Even while a clinical evaluation may shed light on the kind and severity of facial weakness, imaging tests, and electromyography are essential for ruling out other possible explanations and verifying the diagnosis. To guarantee a comprehensive and precise diagnosis, doctors from different specialties—such as neurology and otolaryngology—often need to work together. For those with Bell's palsy, an early diagnosis enables the immediate beginning of suitable therapy, such as corticosteroids, which may improve their prognosis.

CHAPTER FOUR

Treatment Options And Early Intervention For Bell's Palsy

The Value of Prompt Intervention

1. Faster Recovery: One of the most important ways to speed up the healing process is via early intervention. Treating the condition as soon as possible will help restore face function and shorten the time that symptoms last.

2. Diminishing Severity: Prompt action might stop the symptoms from becoming worse. Prompt intervention may reduce the

degree of nerve injury and improve the overall result.

3. Preventing Long-Term Complications: Early intervention for Bell's Palsy reduces the chance of long-term consequences including involuntary muscular movements, irreversible facial paralysis, or other residual disabilities.

Effect on Recuperation:

1. Workouts for the Face: Physical treatment is often advised, and this includes workouts for the face. Starting these workouts early encourages improved muscle tone and prevents muscular atrophy, which contributes to a more thorough recovery.

2. Neurological Rehabilitation: Retraining face muscles and enhancing coordination by early intervention with neurological rehabilitation procedures may lead to a more thorough recovery.

Keeping Complications at Bay:

1. Bell's palsy may impair the afflicted side's ability to seal their eyes, which can cause dryness and possible injury. Early treatments involve protecting the eye with eye patches, ointments, or artificial tears to avoid problems such as corneal abrasions.

2. Speech and Swallowing treatment: Early intervention with treatment helps minimize issues linked to speech and swallowing skills when facial weakness impacts these activities.

Drugs:

1. Corticosteroids:

• Goal: Prednisone is one of the corticosteroids that are often administered to treat edema and inflammation around the facial nerve.

• Timing: Usually given during the first 72 hours of the beginning of symptoms, early in the course of Bell's palsy.

• Impact: Research indicates that when given quickly, corticosteroids may increase the likelihood of a full recovery.

2. Antiviral Medication:

• Goal: Although the effectiveness of antiviral drugs such as acyclovir is debatable, they are sometimes used to treat viral infections (such as the herpes simplex virus) that may be connected to Bell's palsy.

• Timing: Given in addition to corticosteroids, particularly when a viral etiology is thought to be involved.

3. Additional Supportive Drugs:

• Pain Management: To treat any pain or discomfort related to Bell's Palsy, a doctor may give analgesics or other painkillers.

• Physical treatment: In addition to pharmaceuticals, electrical stimulation, and massage treatment may be used to improve muscular function.

In conclusion, a thorough treatment plan and early intervention are essential for effectively treating Bell's palsy. The course of the disease may be greatly impacted by prompt pharmaceutical delivery, especially corticosteroids when combined with supportive therapy. This can expedite recovery and reduce the likelihood of complications. For individualized guidance and treatment recommendations, always seek the opinion of a healthcare provider.

CHAPTER FIVE

Bell's Palsy Physical Therapy And Rehabilitation

The Function Of Physical Therapy

1. Evaluation and Customized Treatment Programs:

• Based on each patient's unique situation, physical therapists determine the degree of face muscle weakness and create customized therapy programs.

• Examining functional ability, muscular strength, range of motion, and facial symmetry may be part of the first examination.

2. Instruction and Assistance:

• Spreading knowledge of Bell's Palsy, the likelihood of recovery, and the value of early intervention.

• Providing coping mechanisms and emotional support, as facial paralysis may affect one's mental health and sense of self.

Exercises To Tone Your Face Muscles:

1. Strengthening of the Face Muscles:

• Targeted workouts concentrate on strengthening particular face muscles damaged by paralysis.

Lip pursing workouts, cheek lifts, and eyebrow raises are a few examples.

2. Exercises for Range of Motion:

• Exercises that increase the afflicted facial muscles' range of motion, fostering suppleness and avoiding rigidity.

• You may include some gentle facial stretches.

Speech Pathology:

1. Practices for Speaking:

• Speech therapists concentrate on exercises to enhance articulation and pronunciation that are impacted by weakness in the facial muscles.

• Exaggerating facial motions and rehearsing speaking sounds are two possible techniques.

2. Exercises for Swallowing:

• Dealing with swallowing issues that might result from weak muscles.

• Exercises designed specifically to improve the strength and coordination of the swallowing muscles.

Techniques For Rehabilitation:

1. Stretching and Massage:

• Massage Therapy: Light pressure applied to the afflicted face muscles might help relax them, increase blood flow, and lessen tension.

• Stretching Exercises: Maintaining muscular suppleness and preventing contractures are achieved by controlled stretching.

2. Biofeedback:

• Biofeedback is the process of providing visual or aural input on muscle activity via technological monitoring.

• Patients gain conscious control over their muscular function, which helps to increase their strength and coordination.

3. Electrical Induction:

• To activate the muscles of the face, one may use neuromuscular electrical stimulation or transcutaneous electrical nerve stimulation (TENS).

• By doing so, you may encourage muscle reeducation and avoid muscular atrophy.

4. Mirror Counseling:

• Involves projecting symmetrical face motions onto a mirror.

• By encouraging the brain to remodel itself, this approach enhances coordination and motor control.

The goals of physical therapy and rehabilitation, which are essential parts of Bell's Palsy management, are to enhance overall quality of life and recover facial muscle function. Exercises, speech therapy, and rehabilitation methods together provide a thorough strategy to address the particular difficulties this illness presents. A more successful healing process is facilitated by patient education, continuous evaluation, and customized treatment programs. Always seek the counsel of medical specialists for individualized recommendations and direction based on your unique requirements.

CHAPTER SIX

Alternative And Supplemental Medical Practices

For those who have Bell's Palsy, which is characterized by an abrupt, transient weakening or paralysis of the facial muscles, it may be a difficult condition.

While corticosteroids and other traditional medical treatments are often administered, some patients look into complementary and alternative therapies in order to improve their recovery or control their symptoms. Herbal and nutritional supplementation, along with acupuncture, are two common methods in this regard.

Acupuncture:

Evidence and Effectiveness: Acupuncture, an age-old Chinese treatment that involves inserting tiny needles into predetermined body sites, has drawn interest as a possible Bell's palsy treatment. Acupuncture may assist in enhancing facial muscle function and lessen Bell's Palsy symptoms, according to some research. The hypothesis behind acupuncture is that it might promote blood flow and neuron regeneration.

It's important to remember, however, that there is conflicting data on the efficacy of acupuncture in treating Bell's palsy. While some studies have shown good results, others find no discernible difference between acupuncture and a placebo.

Safety Considerations: When administered by qualified and certified professionals, acupuncture is usually regarded as safe. Before deciding to get acupuncture, people with Bell's palsy should use caution and speak with their medical professionals. In order to reduce the danger of infection or other consequences, it is important to make sure the acupuncturist is certified and adheres to health and safety regulations.

Supplements Containing Herbs And Nutrients:

Possible Advantages: It is thought that a number of dietary and herbal supplements may be advantageous for those who have Bell's palsy. Among them are:

Vitamin B12: Well-known for its function in maintaining the health of nerves, some believe that taking supplements of this vitamin may promote nerve regeneration and alleviate symptoms.

Omega-3 Fatty Acids: Suggested to have anti-inflammatory qualities, omega-3 fatty acids are present in fish oil and certain nuts and may help lessen inflammation linked to Bell's Palsy.

Zinc: Immune system performance and wound healing depend on this mineral. Some people think that taking zinc supplements might help Bell's palsy patients recuperate.

Warnings and Contraindications: Although there may be advantages to using these supplements, prudence is advised:

Drug Interactions: Some supplements may have drug interactions with those used for Bell's Palsy or other medical disorders. It's important to let medical professionals know about any supplements you use.

Dosage and Product Quality: The combination of these two factors might affect how effective supplements are. To find reliable supplement brands and decide the right dose, it's best to speak with a healthcare provider.

Individual Variability: Different people may react differently to supplements. One person's solution may not be another's. It's important to keep an eye out for any negative effects and to speak with a healthcare professional if you have any concerns.

In conclusion, people with Bell's palsy may think about complementary and alternative therapies like acupuncture and herbal/nutritional supplements, but it's important to approach these alternatives conscious of the little and sometimes conflicting data. To make sure that any treatments selected are in line with the overall treatment plan, do not present hazards, and do not conflict with traditional medical practices, it is essential to have open contact with healthcare practitioners.

CHAPTER SEVEN

Handling Psychological And Emotional Difficulties

Bell's palsy may be a difficult illness because of its effects on emotional and psychological health in addition to its physical symptoms. One of the most important aspects of properly treating Bell's Palsy is learning to cope with the emotional and psychological obstacles it presents.

Aspects Emotional Of Bell's Palsy:

Beauty and Self-Respect:

The unexpected development of facial paralysis may have a profound effect on a person's perception of their body and sense of self.

Feelings of self-consciousness and social anxiety might arise from changes in facial appearance.

Communication Challenges:

Communication problems may arise from facial muscle weakness that affects speaking and facial emotions.

Feelings of loneliness, shame, and irritation might arise from this.

Anxiety and Uncertainty:

Bell's palsy is abrupt and unexpected, which might raise concerns about the future and how long the symptoms will last.

Stress levels might rise when there is uncertainty regarding the amount of recovery.

Influence On Mental Well-Being:

Depression

Bell's palsy patients may exhibit signs of depression as a result of the condition's effects on their physical appearance and day-to-day difficulties.

It's possible to experience powerlessness and despair.

Social Detachment:

Withdrawal from social engagements and activities may be a coping mechanism for facial paralysis.

Isolation may aggravate mental health problems and lead to feelings of loneliness.

Anxiety and Exhaustion:

It may be taxing to manage everyday responsibilities and deal with the physical symptoms, which increases stress and exhaustion.

Long-term stress may have a negative impact on mental health.

Adaptive Techniques:

Psychoeducation:

It's critical to comprehend the illness, its causes, and the chances of healing.

Having knowledge makes it easier for people to control expectations and deal with unpredictability.

Therapy & Counseling:

Getting professional therapy or counseling may provide a secure setting for developing coping mechanisms and expressing feelings.

Treating negative thinking patterns may be especially beneficial for those undergoing cognitive-behavioral treatment (CBT).

Techniques for Relaxation and Mindfulness:

Techniques like deep breathing exercises and mindfulness meditation may aid in stress management and enhance emotional health.

These methods may be included in regular activities to provide continuous assistance.

Systems Of Support:

Support from Family and Community:

It is essential to have open lines of contact with friends and family.

Teaching family members about the illness promotes empathy and understanding.

Support Teams:

Participating in a Bell's Palsy support group helps foster a feeling of camaraderie and common experiences.

Developing relationships with others going through comparable struggles might help you feel less alone.

Expert Assistance:

Speaking with medical specialists, such as social workers or psychologists, may provide specialized assistance.

Experts in rehabilitation can help with the creation of daily activity management methods.

People may improve their general well-being and resilience in the face of this disease by attending to the emotional components, getting expert help, and developing a strong support system.

CHAPTER EIGHT
Changes In Lifestyle For Long-Term Health

1. Handling Stress:

Engage in stress-reduction practices like yoga, deep breathing, and meditation.

Since stress may intensify symptoms, stress management is essential to general health.

2. Physical Medicine:

Follow a physical therapist's advice while doing face exercises to help preserve muscle tone and enhance facial movement.

Giving yourself regular, light face massages might help avoid muscular atrophy.

3. Sufficient Sleep:

Make sure you get enough sleep to aid in your general recuperation.

Don't overdo it and allow your body enough time to recover.

4. Eye Health:

Avoid dry eyes by using artificial tears or eye drops, particularly if Bell's Palsy impairs the closure of the eyelids.

To protect the injured eye while you sleep, think about using an eye patch.

The Dietary Guidelines:

1. Anti-Inflammatory Food Plan:

Eat a diet high in fruits, vegetables, and omega-3 fatty acids, which are strong in antioxidants and anti-inflammatory qualities.

Processed meals, sugary snacks, and too much caffeine should be avoided or limited.

2. Drinking plenty of water

Drink enough water to promote general health and speed up the healing process.

Sufficient hydration encourages healing and preserves the flexibility of the skin.

3. Consumption of vitamins and minerals:

Make sure your diet is well-balanced and contains enough vitamins and minerals, particularly zinc, vitamin B12, and vitamin B6. These nutrients are critical for nerve health and function.

Examine supplements with the advice of a medical practitioner.

Protecting And Taking Care Of The Face:

1. Keeping Complications at Bay:

Shield the afflicted side of your face from the sun, wind, and very cold temperatures.

When it's chilly outside, wear a hat or scarf, and when it's sunny outside, use sunscreen with a high SPF.

2. Skincare Advice:

To avoid dryness and irritation of the skin, keep the afflicted region clean and moisturized.

Employ gentle, hypoallergenic cleansers and moisturizers to steer clear of any allergens.

3. Eye Defense:

To keep the afflicted eye from becoming dry and irritated, use lubricating eye drops.

Think about using sunglasses to shield your eyes from wind and intense sunshine.

4. Dental Health:

Maintaining proper dental hygiene might help avoid issues with drooling and difficulties swallowing.

Frequent dental examinations are necessary to treat any problems with the regulation of muscles in the mouth.

It's crucial to remember that these lifestyle changes are an addition to medical therapies, and people with Bell's palsy should speak with medical specialists for tailored guidance based on their unique requirements and conditions.

CHAPTER NINE

Recurrence Prevention And Upcoming Issues

The rapid development of facial muscular weakness or paralysis, generally on one side of the face, is the hallmark of Bell's palsy. Even though most instances end on their own, it is crucial to avoid recurrence and think about long-term treatment in order to ensure the well-being of those who are impacted by this illness.

Methods For Preventing Recurrence:

Changes in Lifestyle:

Handling Stress: Bell's Palsy has been connected to both the development and worsening of stress. Recurrence may be avoided by using stress-reduction strategies including yoga, meditation, and mindfulness.

Healthy Diet: Anti-inflammatory foods included in a well-balanced diet may help maintain the general health of the facial nerves. It is essential to consume enough vitamins and minerals, especially those that promote nerve function.

Physical Medicine:

Exercises for the Face: Regularly doing exercises for the face will assist in enhancing muscle tone and stop recurrence. Physical therapists may lead people through exercises that are customized to meet their requirements.

Management of Medication:

Antiviral Drugs: Antiviral drugs may be recommended to lower the chance of recurrence in Bell's Palsy situations when viral infections (such as herpes simplex) are linked to the condition.

Corticosteroids: To reduce inflammation and speed up healing, short-term corticosteroid therapy during the first episode may also be taken into consideration.

Extended-Term Administration:

Frequent Examinations:

Neurological Evaluation: Regular neurological evaluations may assist in tracking the general well-being of the facial nerve and early identification of any possible recurrence indicators.

Ongoing Rehabilitation: To preserve ideal facial muscle function, people may find it helpful to see a physical therapist on a regular basis.

Support for Education:

Patient education may enable patients to take proactive steps to avoid recurrence by providing them with information on Bell's Palsy, its causes, and possible warning signals.

Symptom Recognition: Empowering people to identify symptoms early on enables timely intervention, which may lessen the intensity and length of repeated episodes.

Keeping An Eye On Facial Health:

Self-care Routines:

Bell's palsy may impair eyelid closure, thus wearing the right eye protection is essential to avoiding consequences like corneal abrasions. It could be advised to use protective eyewear and lubricating eye drops.

Oral health and dentistry:

Frequent Dental Checkups: People should schedule routine dental appointments to preserve good oral health since poor facial muscles might impair how well they clean their teeth.

Prospective Advances In The Management Of Bell's Palsy:

Investigations and New Treatments:

Medicines that regulate the immunological Response: Research on medicines that regulate the immunological response is ongoing and has the potential to lessen the severity and recurrence of Bell's Palsy.

Nerve Regeneration: Research-based therapies centered on nerve regeneration might provide viable paths toward sustained healing and lowered recurrence rates.

Patient Involvement and Advocacy:

Engagement in Clinical Trials: Encouraging patients to take part in clinical trials may hasten the creation of novel therapeutic approaches and improve the care of Bell's palsy.

Patient Support Groups: Creating and supporting patient support groups may help people feel more connected to one another, provide insightful perspectives, and promote constant communication between patients, medical professionals, and researchers.

In conclusion, a thorough approach to treating Bell's palsy should take into account the long-term well-being of those afflicted as well as efforts to avoid recurrence in addition to urgent therapy. Emerging treatments in conjunction with ongoing research, patient education, and engagement provide hope for a more successful and patient-centered approach to Bell's palsy management.

Conclusion

In Summary:

To sum up, treating Bell's palsy requires a thorough and all-encompassing strategy that goes beyond only treating its symptoms. People may improve their general well-being in addition to properly managing the disease by using a streamlined solution method. The following main ideas emphasize the crucial components of this strategy:

Early Intervention and Health Care:

Early detection and prompt medical intervention are essential for the treatment of Bell's palsy.

Results may be greatly enhanced by administering corticosteroids and antiviral drugs on time.

Rehabilitation and Physical Therapy:

Regaining muscular control and strength may be facilitated by physical therapy and face exercises.

Individualized rehabilitation methods help patients recover more quickly.

Stress Reduction and Mental Wellness:

It is essential to recognize the emotional toll that Bell's palsy takes.

Using stress-reduction strategies like therapy and mindfulness promotes mental health.

Healthy Eating and Living:

Nerve function and healing are supported by a diet high in vitamins and minerals and well-balanced.

Overall health is enhanced by leading a healthy lifestyle that includes frequent exercise and enough sleep.

Continuous Observation and Investigation:

Consultations with medical specialists on a regular basis guarantee ongoing assessment and modification of the treatment plan.

Long-term health depends on early detection and treatment of any possible problems.

Summary Of Main Ideas:

Early Identification and Determination:

Successful treatment of Bell's palsy depends on early detection of the condition's symptoms and timely medical intervention.

Medical Care:

The cornerstones of medical care are corticosteroids and antiviral drugs, which highlight the need for early intervention.

Physical Medicine:

Physical therapy and face exercises can restore facial muscle function and avoid long-term consequences.

Emotional Health:

The healing process depends on recognizing and treating Bell's palsy's emotional effects.

Diet and Way of Life:

Maintaining a healthy lifestyle in addition to eating well-balanced food helps the body's natural healing processes.

Frequent Monitoring

Ongoing observation and communication with medical professionals guarantee that any new problems are quickly detected and resolved.

Providing People With The Tools For Lifelong Health:

A feeling of agency and accountability for maintaining one's own well-being must be ingrained in people in order to empower them for lifetime health. Important components consist of:

Knowledge and Consciousness:

Giving people knowledge about Bell's palsy promotes comprehension and gives them the ability to make wise choices.

Self-Healing Techniques:

By teaching self-care techniques like stress reduction, a balanced diet, and frequent exercise, people may take an active role in their own healing.

Creating Support Systems:

Helping people deal with the psychological and physical difficulties brought on by Bell's palsy involves encouraging them to get assistance from friends, family, and support groups.

Healthy Habits for Life:

Long-term well-being is ensured by encouraging behaviors that support general health, such as maintaining a balanced lifestyle, frequent exercise, and preventative healthcare measures.

In summary, a reduced-risk strategy for Bell's palsy includes health care, therapy, psychological support, and lifestyle modifications. Giving people the tools they need to take control of their health lays the groundwork for long-term well-being.

THE END